SO OUR KID IS SICK, NOW WHAT?
An Anecdotal Evidence Guide

Joshua LeBreton

SPECIAL THANKS:

To Mark Sisson, who inadvertently taught me to see health and wellness in a whole new way. To Dr. Mark Hyman, who, from afar, helped validate the uncharted concepts I had discovered. And to others like them, who encouraged me to believe that healing is within reach.

To Joelle, my loyal wife, who makes space to follow me, even when she's not sure where we'll end up, and who reminded me not to write this book only for myself.

To the family and friends brave enough to support us before our efforts had fully come to fruition, and to those who helped refine and sharpen these perspectives.

Finally, to my daughter, Julia, who trusted that her daddy wanted the best for her and embraced this journey without losing any of her joy or spark. I'm so proud of you. May this serve as a memoir for the years to come, a reminder of why we do what we do.

PREFACE

I almost didn't write this book, but I had to do something to finally free myself from the grip of desperation this season of life had on my family.

One typical weekday morning in the middle of spring, I realized my two-year-old daughter had developed a small limp. By the weekend, she could hardly walk. Her left knee joint had swollen to the size of a baseball. My wife and I were alarmed, confused, and most of all, scared. She was in real pain, but we had no idea why.

With our first and only child, we were already in unknown territory. So, we went through the motions. We made the calls. We saw the doctors. We followed their chain of command. We ran the tests. It took time, lots of it, and the process was neither cheap nor convenient. We waited, waited some more, and then we traveled.

She would eventually be diagnosed with an inflammatory autoimmune disease called Juvenile Idiopathic Arthritis, and medication was the suggested treatment. This helped us so much that we soon saw remission, but I knew we were dealing with dangerous, symptom-modifying drugs. It wasn't something I could accept long-term. Pharmaceuticals would be part of her story, but I just couldn't see them as the end of it.

Throughout the time before, during, and after the diagnosis, I studied everything I possibly could about my daughter's condition. I had to learn why this was happening to her, because maybe then I could figure out what to do about it. What I found was so convoluted and difficult to follow that I almost lost myself entirely in the pursuit. But what I gathered was simple: the body wants to heal. The body can, in fact, heal itself. It needs our help. It requires resources and must have certain obstacles removed. Our DNA is ancient, and its needs are something society has long ignored and forgotten.

When our daughter achieved her unmedicated remission, it became clear that we are not slaves to disease. We can fight when it shows up, distance ourselves before it arrives, and sometimes even prevent its visit altogether. My goal is to inspire the courage to believe this.

The following suggestions are purely anecdotal, N = 1 evidence, but it's all about moving the master needle, not focusing on the minutiae. I am no scientist nor a healthcare professional, but that didn't stop me from being curious. Our reward was a realistic whole-house-forward approach, not just in sickness, but toward health.

It is our innate responsibility to protect our family from the rising tide of chronic disease. Here's how we did it.

CONTENTS

1.

Everyday Lifestyle

Gut Health

How the outside world meets our inside world means everything. Digestion is where whole-body health begins, but perfection isn't the goal. It's about having a happy, super-strong belly.

The gut is as much ours as it is a living world, the microbiome. Think of it like a zoo. Zoos have walls, animals, a few pests, and a food supply. All are equal. We must build up our walls and care for the animals. If we protect it, it will protect us.

Mealtimes & Overnight Fasting

Nobody should be eating around the clock. Our gut isn't designed to digest for long; it needs consistent breaks.

Choose regular mealtimes and stick with them. Avoid drinking something other than water, snacking, or having anything else outside of those meals. Limit your drinking while eating, but have plenty of water between meals. Arrange mealtimes 3 to 5 hours apart, giving your gut time to finish its job and blood sugar time to settle.

Overnight fasting is a longer break, and when real magic happens. After your last bite of the day, leave at least 12 hours before your first bite the next morning. Plain water is always fine during fasting. This works best with an earlier dinner and a well-timed breakfast. We're not skipping meals, just getting much needed time off.

Sleep

Sleep is the special time when our bodies will truly heal themselves, if we let them. Once digestion is finished and our hormones are at rest, now the body can focus on clearing out waste. It's like going into deep-cleaning mode.

Create a nighttime routine and stick to it. Go to sleep and wake up around the same time every day. Put away screens or apply a red filter to the lights an hour before bedtime. Cool down your room and make it very dark. Avoid sleep aids. Our bodies need 7 to 9 hours of natural, nightly sleep.

Sunlight

Earth is alive because of the sun. While it can be dangerous, it's not our enemy. Spend time with it. Let it touch your skin, without sunblock or sunglasses, but be mindful of the time of day and how long you're exposed.

Notice the morning sunrise, afternoon sun, and the evening sunset. Our internal clocks get lost without these signals.

Exercise

We are made to move, to use our muscles. Movement and muscle remind our bodies to stay alive.

Exercise to build and keep muscle, strengthen bones, lower body fat, reduce stress, and have your gut's microbiome make post-biotic, short-chain fatty acids that help us get fit from the inside out.

RECAP WORDS: *Belly Zoo. Eat, Break. Bedtime. Internal Clock. Movement.*

2.

Nutrition Planning

Water

Drinking clean water is a first floor human need. It's not just a healthy habit, but it is an easy one to adopt.

Since we're all different, the foolproof way to know if you are getting enough water is by checking your urine. If it's too dark, you'll need more. If it is too clear, you are overdoing it. Aim for a light, pale yellow, much like the color of lemonade.

Big & Little Nutrition

The big nutrition three are Proteins, Fats, and Carbohydrates. Protein gets a lot of the praise, Fat tends to be feared, and Carbohydrates are obsessed over.

In my view, protein should be the priority, fat should be eaten freely but with attention to its type, and then carbohydrates, where included, should be chosen mainly for their color and soluble fiber content, not to be confused with insoluble fiber.

A lack of little nutrition, like vitamins and minerals, can cause the body to break down in ways we might not expect. Our bodies rely on these resources to work, and our gut's microbiome needs some too, helping us absorb it all.

Ancestor Foods

The way we eat today is a far cry from how our ancestors did, yet our DNA still belongs to that old world. Our bodies long for what's missing from today's food practices. We are filled with empty eats but starved of nutrition.

If we viewed food the way our ancestors did, we could know a whole foods diet that supports us while still offering plenty of modern flexibility...

Potent-Proteins:

GRASS-FED RED MEATS
PASTURE-RAISED EGGS & POULTRY
WILD FATTY, SHELL, & WHITE FISH
FERMENTED DAIRY
BONE BROTH
ORGAN MEATS

Includes: *★Beef, Bison, ★Deer, Lamb / ★Chicken, ★Duck, Turkey / ★Sockeye Salmon, Sardine / ★Oyster, Shrimp / ★Cod / <u>Plain</u>: ★Cheese, ★Greek Yogurt / ★Beef plus Chicken Bone / Heart, ★Liver.*

★FAVORITES

Proteins aren't meant for energy; our bodies use them as building blocks. Animal proteins tend to have more, while plant-based proteins offer less. But remember, what an animal eats is what they, and then we, become.

Fantastic-Fats:

OLIVE
AVOCADO
TREE NUTS
SEEDS
COCONUT
GRASS-FED ANIMAL FATS

Includes: *Extra Virgin Olive Oil, *Kalamata / *Avocado Oil, *Hass / Dry Roasted/Soaked: *Almond, Hazelnut, *Macadamia, Pecan, *Pistachio, Walnut / Raw/Sprouted: *Cacao plus *Dark Chocolate, Chia, *Cold-Ground Flax, Hemp, *Pumpkin, Sesame, Sunflower / *Coconut: Milk, Oil / *Butter, *Cream, Ghee, *Tallow.

*__FAVORITES__

Lean on monounsaturated fats (MUFA), enjoy some saturated fats (SFA), and be mindful with polyunsaturated fats (PUFA).

MUFAs are the least controversial, while SFAs are a hotter topic, but any risks with saturated fats largely depend on sourcing and overall amounts. PUFAs, on the other hand, are less stable and prone to going rancid, contributing to chronic inflammation. However, some PUFAs, like the Omega-3s found in fatty fish, are essential for balancing inflammation.

Clever-Carbohydrates:

NON-STARCHY & ROOT VEGETABLES
LOW-GLYCEMIC FRUITS & SQUASHES
ASIAN MUSHROOMS
BEANS & LEGUMES
PSEUDOCEREALS

Includes: Cooked: *Artichoke, *Asparagus, *Broccoli, *Brussels Sprout, Cabbage, *Cauliflower, *Leafy Greens, *Seaweed, *Beet, Carrot, *Cassava, Konjac, *Sweet Potato / *Apple, *Apricot, *Blackberry, *Dark Sweet Cherry, *Kiwi,

Papaya, Pear, *Raspberry, *Strawberry, *Wild Blueberry, Butternut, *Cucumber, *Pumpkin, *Spaghetti / Cooked: *Lion's Mane, Oyster, *Shiitake / Cooked: *Black Bean, Chickpea, Lentil, *Pea, *Pinto / Cooked: Amaranth, *Buckwheat, Quinoa.

*FAVORITES

Carbohydrates provide a fuel, but too much can cause harmful blood sugar levels. The body will defend itself, which can lead to insulin resistance, weight gain, and worse. Poor choices encourage bad cholesterol ratios, fatty liver, gut dysbiosis, high blood pressure, and lousy sleep, while raising the risk of dementia, diabetes, heart disease, stroke, and more.

Except for athletes, starches and sugars from any carbohydrate should be limited, but their pre-biotic soluble fiber is what feeds our gut's microbiome.

Fortifying-Ferments:

LIVE-CULTURED DAIRY & VEGETABLES

Includes: <u>Plain</u>: *Cottage Cheese, *Kefir, plus *Yogurt / Kimchi, *Miso, Nattō, *Pickles, *Sauerkraut, Tempeh.

*****FAVORITES**

Full of pro-biotic bacteria, these add animals to our belly zoo.

Smart-Spices & Sweeteners:

Includes: *Apple Cider Vinegar, Black Peppercorn, *Blackstrap Molasses, *Ceylon Cinnamon, Cloves, *Coconut Aminos, Coconut Sugar, Cumin, Date Sugar, Date Syrup, Fenugreek, *Garlic, *Ginger, *Lemon Juice, *Maple Syrup, Monk Fruit, *Non-Fortified Nutritional Yeast, Onion, *Raw Honey, *Sea Salt, Turmeric.

*****FAVORITES**

Moderate amounts carry electrolytes and flavor, while delivering powerful health benefits.

Miscellaneous-Menu:

Includes: *Coffee / *Green & Herbal Tea.*

*FAVORITES

Rich in antioxidants, flavonoids, and polyphenols, these are best enjoyed along with meals, where they can be dressed as desired. If having before, between, or after mealtimes, do so less often and without stir-ins.

———

These foods can become everything from condiments, dressings, and sauces to baked goods, breads, chips, crackers, flours, nut butters, pastas, tortillas, and other processed-food lookalikes.

Plan, prep, cook, store, and eat in simple ways. This builds a strategy you can repeat again and again, helping you avoid feeling overwhelmed. Simple is easy, and easy still gets lasting results.

Supplements

Diet and lifestyle always come first. There's a relationship between food and the body that supplements can't replace, though they can offer extra support.

Includes: *Whole Food Multivitamin with B-Vitamins, D3, plus K2 **/** Marine DHA & EPA Omega-3s **/** Grass-Fed Bovine Collagen Peptides **/** Magnesium Glycinate.*

Take them with balanced meals that include big and little nutrition foods. Be careful with additives, dosing, quality, and realize that with these, less is more.

Treat Days

Anything within reason goes on treat days, as they're not for the body but for the soul. They help us connect socially, give us freedom, and keep us from daydreaming about the foods we limit.

Looking after our health 85% of the time makes space to loosen up for that leftover 15%, but everyone tolerates this uniquely. Eat well most days, make treats the exception, and adapt it to suit you.

RECAP WORDS: *Hydrate. Real Foods. Extra Support. Fun Foods.*

3.

Healthy Fears

Tap Water

Tap water is legally safe, but what our bodies have to filter out of it is far from safe. Chlorine, fluoride, forever chemicals, heavy metals, pesticides, and plastics are just the tip of the iceberg, and disposable plastic bottles only add to the problem.

Look for a water filter that tackles these concerns without stripping away all the minerals. The best option is a whole-house system, but at the very least, we should filter the water we use for cooking, drinking, and eating.

Ultra-Processed Foods

Ultra-Processed Foods are not food. Food feeds our body; UPF's only fill it. Processing can turn nuts into nut butter and even milk into a yogurt, but ultra-processing makes the original food almost unrecognizable. This makes us sick but earns big companies millions of dollars.

UPF's come loaded with refined colors, flavors, flours, gums, high-fructose syrups, preservatives, sodium, starches, sugars, sweeteners, along with PUFA vegetable oils like canola, corn, cottonseed, peanut, rapeseed, rice bran, safflower, soybean, sunflower, and more.

These hide behind plant-based meats, milks, and cheeses. It's in energy drinks, juices, protein shakes, snack bars, and sodas. They're found in processed meats, fast food, salad dressings, and a lot of what's bagged, bottled, boxed, or canned at the grocery store. They're even in our infant formula and baby foods. Over time, they slowly but surely age and ruin us.

Taboo Topics

Grains:

Grains are where the famously feared gluten is found, mostly in wheat, barley, and rye, including their flours. For those sensitive, even cross-contact with these proteins can trigger a reaction to what would otherwise be safe.

At its worst, gluten is a gut wall shredder. Even at its best, it is only partially digested. No one handles gluten perfectly. Along with similar pieces in other grains, it can cause more problems than it's worth. Including grains in the diet should come with caution.

Non-gluten whole grains with benefits worth considering, carefully, include cooked corn, millet, oats, and rice.

Dairy:

Milk, especially when fermented, can be part of a healthy diet. Some of us have issues with dairy, often related to casein (a protein) or lactose (a carbohydrate). Symptoms from either are usually not subtle, but we have options.

If casein is an issue, look for A2 dairy, which more closely resembles human breast milk. Goat and sheep milk are naturally high in A2 beta-casein, but we can identify cows that share in this too.

If lactose is a problem, fermentation removes nearly all of it while also twisting the milk proteins, making them slightly different from liquid milk.

Milk fats tend to cause issues far less often, but what an animal eats and is exposed to will always influence the quality of its milk.

Soy:

For whole soybeans, fermentation is just as useful as it is with dairy. It turns a potential problem food into one worth a second look.

Nightshades:

Nightshade fruits and vegetables, such as bell peppers, chili peppers, eggplant, tomatoes, and white potatoes, fall into a bit of a gray area. They can be sneakily inflammatory for some, while no bother to others.

Medicines:

The use of medication in our society is out of control. Every medicine comes with a tradeoff; none are innocent. Our bodies process all things the same way.

Antibiotic overuse is one of the bigger threats to gut health. They can tear down strong guts but will destroy a weakened one.

Organic & Non-GMO Foods

Organic food is not automatically health food. There are more rules. It's safer than most conventional animal and crop farming because we skip much of the antibiotic, herbicide, hormone, pesticide, and radiation use, while caring more for the soil where these foods are grown.

An organic apple beats a conventional one, but an organic chip or cracker isn't always a healthy choice. Some things are important to buy organic and worth considering, but organic food is not always necessary.

GMO foods are born in a lab, usually made to withstand heavy farming chemicals. Learn which foods are currently GMOs, why, and what products label themselves as Non-GMO. Organic foods can never be a GMO.

Home Cooking

With oils like avocado, coconut, and extra virgin olive oil, along with grass-fed animal fats such as butter, ghee, and tallow, there's no need to consider heat-sensitive, ultra-processed polyunsaturated seed and vegetable oils in our kitchens. Still, learn the rancid points of these stable cooking fats to prevent turning what is healthy into something harmful.

Cooking low and slow, with heat and time, makes for a safer plate of food. Avoiding non-stick, chemical-coated pans, pots, and surfaces helps us steer clear of cooking toxins into our food. Ditching plastics in kitchen utensils, cutting boards, and other tools decreases our chemical exposure. Heat and plastics aren't a safe mix.

RECAP WORDS: *Filtered Water.*
Fake Foods. Bugaboos. Safer Foods.
Heat.

4.

Paying Attention

Catch Everything

Most things that aren't good for many are usually not great for anyone, but sometimes something healthy for the majority can be harmful to a few. Catch every symptom, whether it's a sniffle, cough, joint pain, gas, skin issue, swelling, sneeze, reflux, fatigue, headache, bellyache, diarrhea, constipation, or anything similar.

The body is always speaking. Listen closely, trust your instincts, and connect the dots. Your outsides are a reflection of your insides. Keep track of it.

Ingredient Lists

Today's processed products are not anything like what our great-grandparents used. Whether it's with candles, cleaning supplies, personal hygiene, or food, be an ingredients list investigator. Read them all, often, and no matter what. If you spot something you wouldn't put in a kitchen or bathroom yourself, or if the list seems endless, just put it back.

Nutrition Facts labels are helpful for finding big and even little nutrition details, but it's in the ingredient lists that true colors come out. Opt for simple products with fewer ingredients, because we are what we smell, taste, and touch.

Mindset

Don't be afraid, feel empowered. We can only control what's controllable, but it's up to us to figure out exactly what that is. Be intentional. Think outside the box. Problem-solve, stay disciplined, and above all, be patient with your progress.

Never take health for granted, life can change in an instant. Try routines and systems until they are new weekly habits. Put effort into building a structure rigid enough to keep your family safe, but still flexible enough to enjoy life. Teach your children the importance of choosing a healthy lifestyle. Make it a family value. It's the only way to win this race against chronic disease. Lead by example. It's not just about reducing what we are doing; it's about adding what's been missing.

Cherish the cheerleaders who support your efforts, but be understanding with those who won't. We all fear change. We are creatures of habit. The problem is, our habits are all wrong, and it's time to switch paths. Believe in yourself and your family, and take it one step at a time. Work with what you have, find your groove. Don't make excuses, create solutions. Be a cycle-breaker, and you'll never regret it!

RECAP WORDS: *Subtle Signs. Modern Things. Attitude.*

NOTES

_____

_____

_____

_____

_____

_____

_____

_____

_____

_____

_____

_____

_____

_____

_____

_____

_____

_____

About The Author

With roots as a creative arts professional, a naturally investigative mindset, and an obsessively curious nature, *Joshua LeBreton*, now a devoted dad, is forced to channel all his solution-oriented focus toward helping his daughter heal from a seemingly incurable inflammatory autoimmune disease diagnosis, born from pure parental desperation to protect.

www.ingramcontent.com/pod-product-compliance
Lightning Source LLC
Chambersburg PA
CBHW060529280326
41933CB00014B/3119